Survival Guide:

20 Skills that Will Keep You Safe In The Wilderness

Table of content

Introduction

What would you do if you are travelling on a plane and suddenly it crashes on an isolated island in the midst of the Pacific Ocean? Surviving in such a situation seems like the most complicated thing on earth. Understanding that you are trapped in a place that is full of unforeseen dangers, without any shelter or food can be quite mind-numbing for any person. But one thing that you must not forget is that surviving in such situation is definitely *possible* if you brace yourself for the complications that you might encounter in the wilderness. This book is a complete and comprehensive guide on how to survive in such a place and keep yourself alive until the help arrives.

After you are left in the wilderness, the first step you have to take is to find a safe and secure shelter where you can seek refuge from the predators until the help arrives. The second chapter of this book will provide you with the details that will help you find a shelter. The third chapter of this book is a complete guide on how to find food and drinking water in order to satisfy your thirst and hunger.

You must also understand that in order to survive in the wilderness, you must not only learn the necessary skills but you must also gain a complete control of your mind and emotional outbursts. Surviving in the complicated conditions of the wilderness is no doubt a tough thing but one can fulfill this task by keeping control of himself. The fourth chapter of this book highlights the skills to understand the dangerous situations that you might encounter in the wilderness and how to keep yourself alive during those situations.

"Wilderness Survival Guide: 20 Skills that Will Get You Out Alive" is not only a book but it is your only hope during the life-threatening situations in the wilderness.

Chapter 1- Understanding basic survival skills: How to plan for survival in the wilderness?

Nobody can predict when a catastrophe is going to hit or when he/she will be left alone to survive in the wilderness. Learning to take care of yourself and surviving in the wilderness is not a simple thing. There are many points that need to be covered under this topic. When you learn that you have to survive in the wilderness then there are many questions that might appear in your mind. First of all, you need to understand and plan the survival strategies that are necessary for your survival. You also make the necessary preparations for your survival because having useful items along with you in the wilderness is going to make your survival easy.

In this chapter, we will be covering three necessary skills for devising strategies and making preparations to survive in the wilderness.

Skill # 1-Planning the Survival Strategies

Before planning for the survival strategies, one must keep his/her mind alert. Because planning for a survival strategy is nothing but recognizing the survival options that are available to you in this wild and dangerous area. Planning for the survival means that you have to find hope in the hopeless situation.

Planning strategies might include all those acts or items that will keep you alive in the wilderness. For instance, if you are left alone in a hilly area where you are trapped inside a house due to continuous snowfall then you have to point out all the necessary items that will help you feed yourself, keep you warm and healthy until the snowfall stops and you can restore your access to the world.

If you constantly go on adventurous trips, then you must also keep a little survival kit or bag with you. This kit must be equipped with all the necessary weapons, life-saving items and medicines that might come useful to you if you are thrown into a tough situation. While preparing a survival kit, you must keep in mind all those situations that you might encounter while your stay in the wilderness.

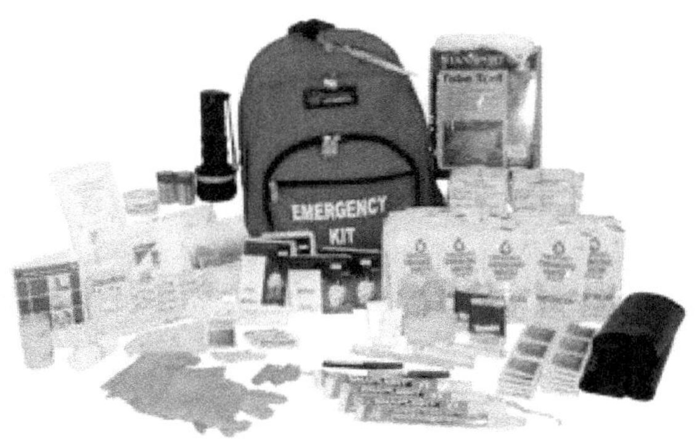

http://www.edisastersystems.com/store/images/D/d-3.jpg

You might face severely cold or hot weather, you might have to light up fire to cook food or keep predators away or you might need to treat yourself with a disinfectant after getting wounded. So you must keep every necessary item with you.

Skill #2-Preparing the Necessary Gear Items

If you are confused about what type of survival kit you must get then you must get the one that can easily be carried around, is water-proof and spacious enough to accommodate all of your survival items. When it comes to the necessary gear items that you must include in your survival kit then you must include all the necessary medicines along with the items used for first aid. You must also include the items used to initiate a fire, tablets or drops used for water purification, a compass, candle and a torch, knife, matches, blanket, and items used for the purpose of signaling.

Skill # 3-Understanding the Medical Necessities

As mentioned above, you must also include a vast range of medicines and other medical items in your survival kit. You must also take complete care of your health and instantly treat any health issue that occurs during your stay in the wilderness. You must drink at least 7-8 liters of water per day in small portions because dehydration might lead you to severe illness. In order to stay healthy, you must also take care of your personal hygiene and keep the surrounding area, especially your shelter clean.

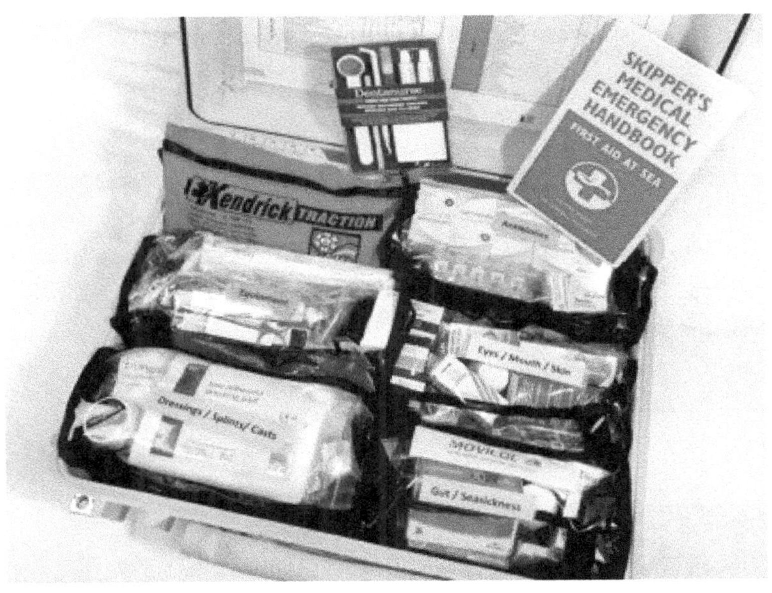

https://www.msos.org.uk/images/
medical_support_offshore_medical_kits_2.jpg

Chapter 2- Skills for seeking shelter in the wilderness

After being left alone in the wilderness, the first and most important step that one must take is to seek refuge inside a reliable shelter. Shelters are very important with respect to security and protection against the dangers of wilderness. Shelter provides you complete protection from the attack of poisonous insects, harsh weathers, and predators. Need for the shelter is usually termed as the primary need but it can be shifted to the second or third number depending on the circumstances of your environment.

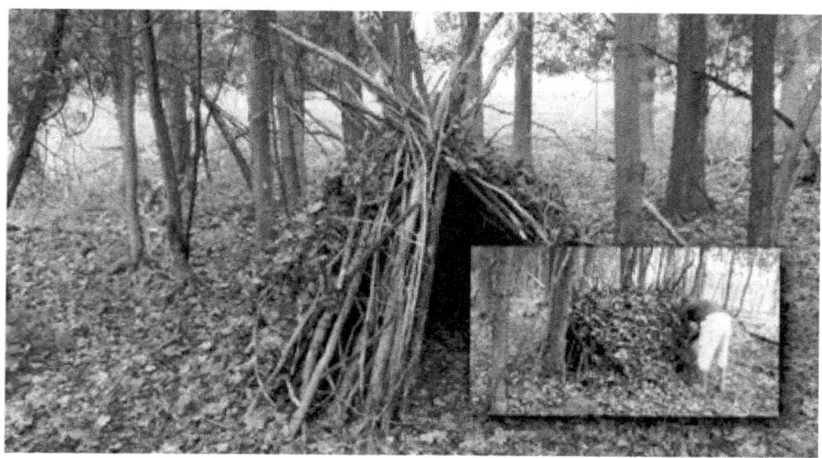

https://i.ytimg.com/vi/royHZdSmorY/maxresdefault.jpg

Skill #4- Finding the Perfect Shelter

Whenever you create a shelter for yourself, you must keep in mind not to create it in a huge size. If the shelter is huge then it might not keep you warm in the chilling weather and will also catch the attention of dangerous animals.

Before creating a shelter in the wilderness, you must observe some of the important things with great care:

- Your environment or your luggage possesses all the basic necessities to create a shelter.

- The location of the shelter must be straight enough to provide you with a comfortable lying area.

- The location for shelter must be situated in a concealed area so it might not catch attention of the predators.

- Location must be safe from the poisonous insects and also possesses paths for escape if the predator attacks.

- You must take care not to select the shelter location right in the way of rock sliding while residing in the mountain areas.

- You must also take care to stay away from the areas with water bodies in order to avoid any damage from the coercive floods.

Another thing that you must understand is that the requirements for the perfect shelter are different in cold areas and hot areas. If you are residing in a hot area for instance a tropical jungle then you might need to get a shelter that is airy, cool, near the water and insect-free. On the other hand, if you are residing in a cold or hilly area then you might be seeking for a shelter that keeps you secure and warm and also provides you an access to the sunlight.

Skill #5-Securing Your Shelter

Finding a perfect shelter for yourself is one thing but securing it against the dangers of the nature is totally a different thing. In order to secure your shelter, you must create a shelter that is strong enough to protect you from harshness of the weather and you must create it in a way that it keeps you safe from the other physical dangers.

While creating a shelter you must build the one that cannot be pointed out due to its perfect blend with the environment. You must also keep the silhouette of your shelter at the lowest possible position. Keeping the shelter in deformed shape or providing it a rough look will also help avoiding the attention of the predators. Again, you must not create a huge shelter but try to keep it as small as comfortably possible. Last but not the least; you must create shelter in an isolated area in order to stay safe from the horrors of the nature.

Chapter 3- Skills for finding basic necessities

Four necessary skills will be discussed in this chapter including the skills to find water, food, light fire and how to feed yourself on wild plants.

Skill #6-Keeping Yourself Hydrated

Keeping yourself hydrated is one of the biggest complications of staying in the wilderness. How can you keep yourself hydrated if you are unable to find purified drinking water? But in order to survive in the wilderness one must learn the tactics to access clean drinking water during his/her stay in the wilderness. Drinking water is very important; an average human can survive up to three days without drinking water but after that, the situation will get worse. So instead of waiting for the third day to arrive, one must start searching for water as soon as possible.

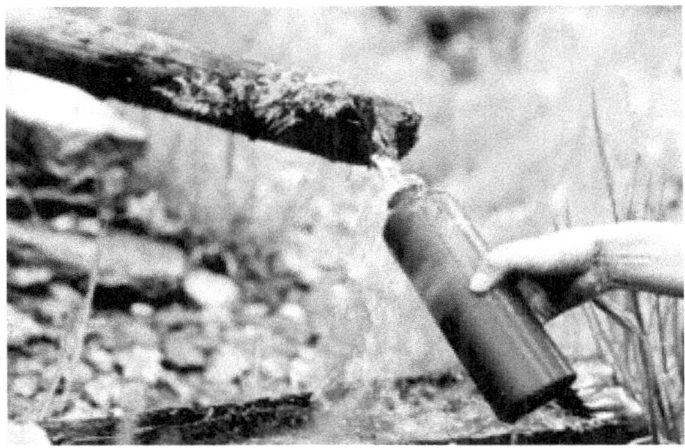

http://www.offthegridnews.com/wp-content/uploads/2014/06/water-wilderness-safely-istock-400x266.jpg

First of all, you need to find a nearby source of water and then purify that water in order to turn it into drinking water. If you are in an area where you can gain access to running stream, then this source is much better than all the other sources of water. Although running stream is not 100% safe as it might contain bacteria for various illnesses but still it's much better and reliable.

If you are not able to find any source of water but you discover the presence of dew on the leaves and flower petals then you must, without any delay, suck in this dew after collecting it on a piece of cloth. Following this step will also help in keeping you alive. Keeping track of the birds might also lead you towards the nearby source of water as birds also drink water in order to quench their thirst.

After finding the water you must learn to purify it before drinking. For this purpose, you can use the water purifying tablets or you can boil it in a pot for three to five minutes after you have lighted the fire.

Skill #7-Building a Fire

Building fire is also very important as not only will it keep you warm but it will also keep the dangerous animals away. So in order to build fire, you must get access to lots of coal or pieces of dry wood. You need to light up the fire before the sunset because lighting a fire will seem more difficult after the sunlight has vanished. Building a fire is extremely important even if you think that the weather is too hot for a fire.

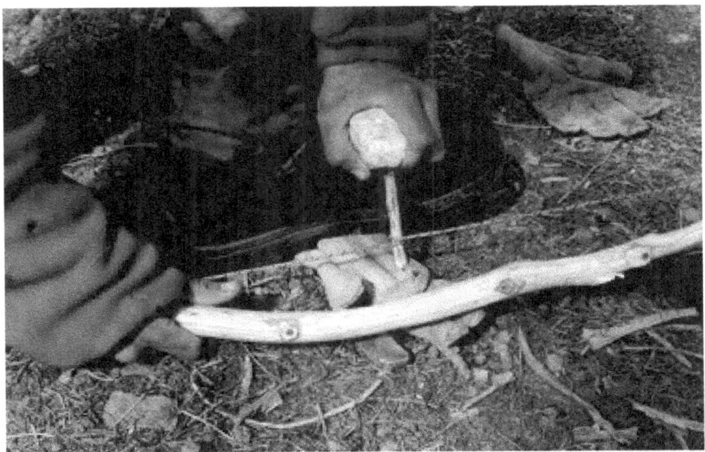

http://survival-mastery.com/wp-content/uploads/2015/02/Starting-a-fire.jpg

The first step that you need to take in order to light a fire is to accumulate three to four piles of dry wood in a reasonable size so you can keep the fire alive throughout the night. If you are unable to gain access to dry wood in the wilderness, then you can also light the fire with the help of the dried dung or tree bark. After lighting the fire, when the fire starts blistering with complete power then you can also add other tree items to fuel the fire. Keeping the fire high might help you in signaling for help because high fire also releases a lot of smoke in the air. You must never light the fire near the trees; instead try to light it in a clearing.

Skill #8-Searching for Food

After you have secured a shelter and found drinking water for yourself, you need to look for the food. Finding food in the wilderness is not an easy task as you have to strive hard to get hold of it.

You must understand that in the wilderness you might find various food items that might be poisonous for you. For instance, some of the mushrooms do look delicious but they are extremely poisonous, so do try to search for healthy and safe food. During your search for food in the wilderness, you must never worry about the taste of the food; instead you must concentrate on the nutrients that will be provided by the wild food.

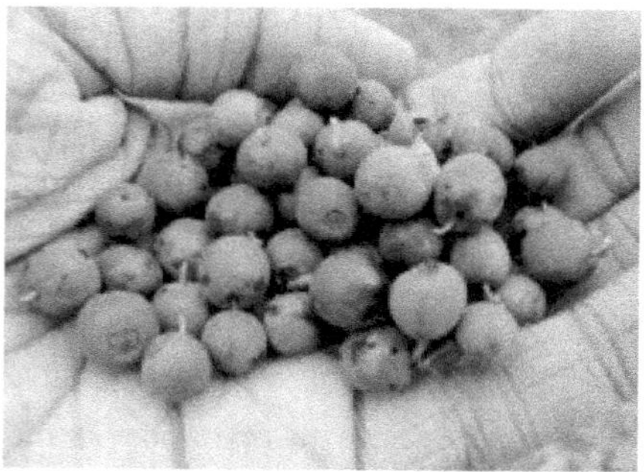

http://www.camptrip.com/wp-content/uploads/2011/04/blueberries_m-300x225.jpg

Instead of going for wild herbs, you must concentrate on fulfilling your food requirements from the insects and animals. At first the thought of eating an insect might make you vomit but insects, without any doubt, are the safest food items in the wilderness.

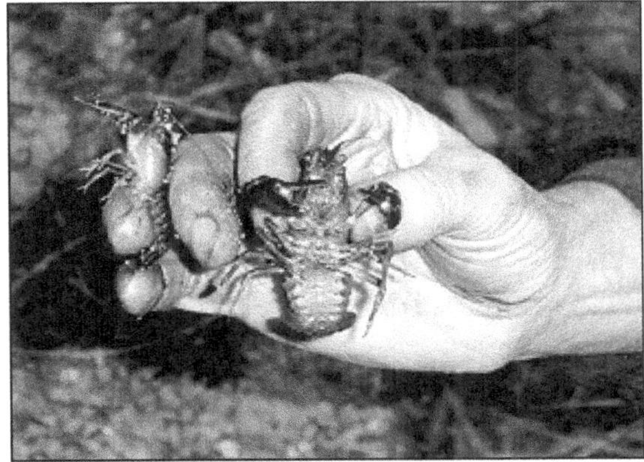

http://www.primitiveways.com/Image3/wilderness_skills13.jpg

Insects are very nutritious as they contain proteins in quite abundance. But here you must keep in mind that not all insects are included in the list of "eatable insects". Some of the insects that are not meant for eating are:

- Adult insects

- Biting insects

- Insects with sting

- Hairy insects

- Insects with bright colors

- Insects with strong odor

- Caterpillars

- Mosquitoes

- Ticks

- Spiders

- Flies

The eatable insects include:

- Grass hopper-in cooked form

- Beetles-in cooked form

- Ants

- Termites

- Grubs

- Worms

If you dwell near the river then you can also eat raw fish in order to satisfy your hunger.

Skill #9-Feeding Yourself on Wild Plants

Plants can also fulfill your need for hunger but the issue with plants is that most of them are poisonous. So in order to satisfy your hunger with plants, you need to understand the nature and effects of the wild plants available in your surrounding area. Bear in mind never to confuse the identification of a wild plant because a single mistake in identifying the plant can mean a matter of life and death. Poison Hemlock is a deadly plant but most of the people reached death after identifying it as wild parsnips.

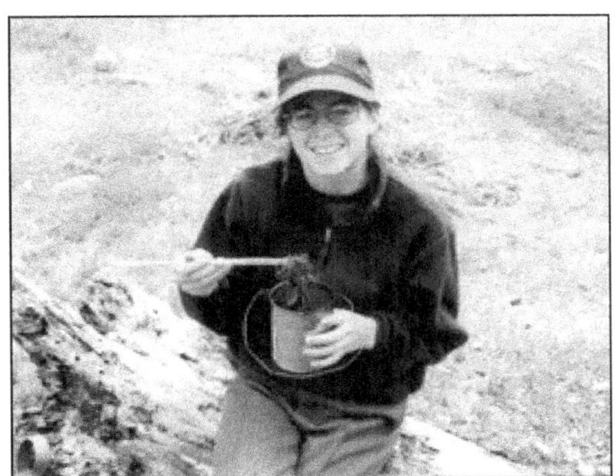

http://www.primitiveways.com/Image3/wilderness_skills56.jpg

If you are stuck in an alien place and don't know much about the plants of that area, then by minding few important points you can easily gain access to eatable plants. If you collected plants from impure water, then you must boil them before eating. Never eat fungus-infested fruits. If you have gotten hold of bitter plants, then you must boil them in the water several times before eating them. If you collected plants from the outer area of a building, then you must deeply wash them before eating as such plants might contain the effects of pesticides.

Protecting yourself against the unforeseen dangers of the wilderness is not an easy task. In this chapter we are going to discuss the three skills of recognizing the dangers in different situations and methods to cope with these dangers.

Skill #10-Understanding the Dangerous Plants

Poisonous plants are extremely dangerous and can provide you harm in many different ways. In order to survive in the wilderness, you must have a complete knowledge about the types of dangerous plants and their harmful effects.

Poisonous plants can easily harm you if you ate it after mistaking it for an eatable plant. If the person comes into contact with a poisonous plant, then he will also receive the dangerous effects of these plants in the form of skin rashes or allergies. Poisonous plants can also harm you through their pollens. If you smell a poisonous pretty flower while mistaking it for a harmful plant, then this act can also put you into extremely painful situation.

You must keep in mind that the poisonous effects of every plant are different from one another. For instance, some of the plants won't incur poisonous effects until you come into contact with these plants on a regular basis. While on the other hand, there are also some plants that are so poisonous that even touching them for a second can cause instant death. Here we must also keep in mind that physical condition of a person also depends on the level of poisoning effects that he/she might receive from the plants. Some people possess extremely sensitive bodies and hence get instant allergic reactions by coming into contact with particular plants.

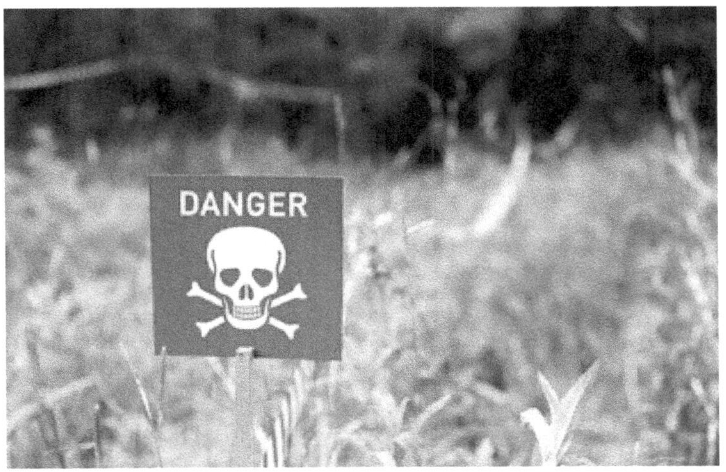

http://media.mnn.com/assets/images/2016/02/danger-sign-plants.jpg

There are different myths about the tests for the poisonous plants and most of them are false. For instance, people usually believe that if the wild plants are boiled in the water before eating them then their poison gets washed away. This concept is false as most of the poisonous plants don't shed their poison even after getting boiled. There is also a myth about the color of the plants. According to this myth, if the plant is red in color then it is definitely poisoned. This myth is also not true as most of the red plants are safe and eatable. Some of the people are also of the opinion that if a person is trying to survive in the wilderness then he/she must keep an eye on the animals feeding on different plants. The plants eaten by the animals are safe for eating. This concept is also false as the digestive system of animals is totally different from that of humans. If an animal doesn't get poisoned by a plant won't mean that it will have similar effect on the humans.

Skill # 11-Protection against Dangerous Animals

Getting attacked by a brutal animal or a flesh-eating insect is one of the biggest fears of staying in the wilderness. You must create your shelter in a hidden, deformed manner so the dangerous animals won't get trace of your presence in the wilderness.

You must also be aware about the types of animals and insects that might be present in the area you are living. Another care that you must take is to dispose off your food remains properly so the animals won't come towards you after catching the smell of the food.

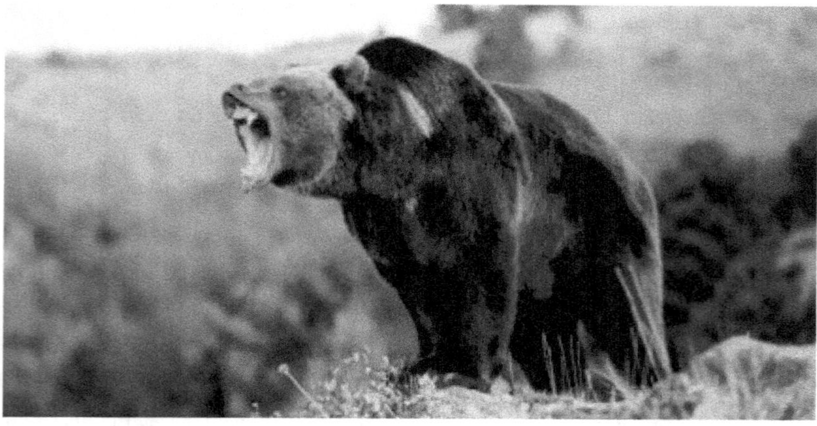

http://img1.rnkr-static.com/list_img_v2/6453/366453/870/tips-for-encountering-5-dangerous-animals-u3.jpg

In some situations, small-sized reptiles or insects are more life threatening than the large-sized animals. In any case, you must try to avoid coming into contact with insects like spiders, scorpions, ticks, bees, centipedes, hornets, millipedes and wasps. The best way to avoid getting attacked by these insects is to keep your shelter and your clothes clean. You must also dust your beddings every morning and at night before bedtime in order to make sure there are no spiders in your bed.

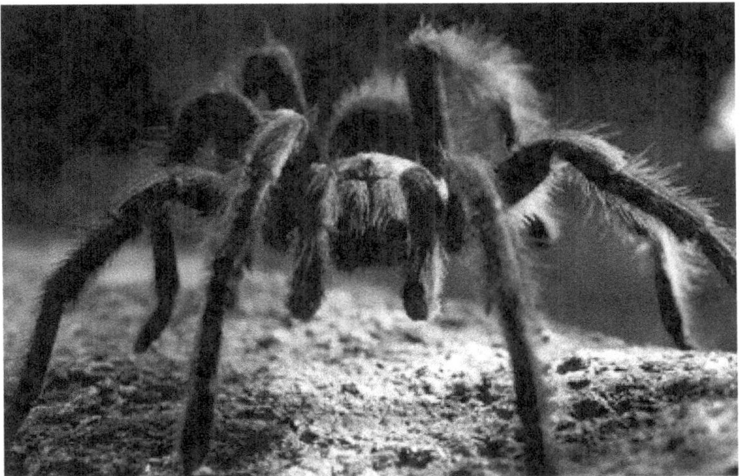

https://usercontent2.hubstatic.com/5476557_f520.jpg

You must take great care if you are allergic to the venom of the wasp because the sting of a wasp and the similar flying insects can be very painful for you and due to your allergies, the venom can also cause your instant death.

Although bats are also termed as dangerous reptiles but in fact few of the bat species are harmful for the humans. The real blood-sucking bats are usually found in the areas of South America, so you don't need to fear them unless you are living in this area.

When it comes to snakes, you must try to avoid all sorts of snakes because you might never know which of them are poisonous and which are harmless. While residing in the wilderness, you must walk carefully and keep a stick with you at all times. If you are picking up plants, vegetables or wild fruits for your food then you must first hit them with a stick to make sure there isn't any snake near them.

Skill #12-Extracting Weapons from Your Surroundings

Whether you are going on an adventure or any business trip, you must always keep some weapons in your bag/purse such as knife, cutter or a lighter. After being stuck in a wilderness, you must always keep these weapons with you because you might never know that when will you come into contact with a predator.

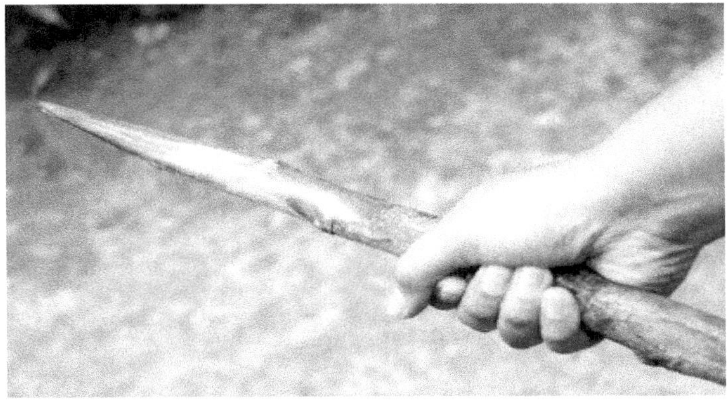

Sometimes it also happens that you suddenly get stuck in the wilderness and you don't even possess a small-sized cutter to protect yourself. In such a situation, you need to keep yourself calm and think about extracting weapons from your surroundings. For instance, you can create a club for yourself from a thick branch of any tree and combine it with a sharp stone in order to provide it the shape of an axe. If you don't have a knife with you then you can also create a knife with the help of a sharp stone. You can also create splinters with the bones of big animals such as goats, bulls, sheep, dead tiger or a deer. All you need to do is to hit that bone with a strong rock in order to break it into splinters. Do keep in mind that you can always sharpen your stone knife or bone splinters by rubbing them against a rock.

Chapter 4- Skills for surviving in different situations

In this chapter, we are going to discuss eight skills to survive in different situations and different environments.

Skill #13-Beating the Heat in Desert Areas

Surviving in the desert areas is not an easy task because intense heat and lack of drinking water are two of the biggest enemies that you will face in the desert. In order to survive in the desert, you must understand that due to elevated external temperature, you body will demand more water so you will need to drink more water. But unfortunately finding drinking water in the desert is something very difficult. You must search for an oasis and in the meanwhile you must try to stay as much away from the sun as possible. If you sit on the ground, then first place your bag on the ground and then sit on it.

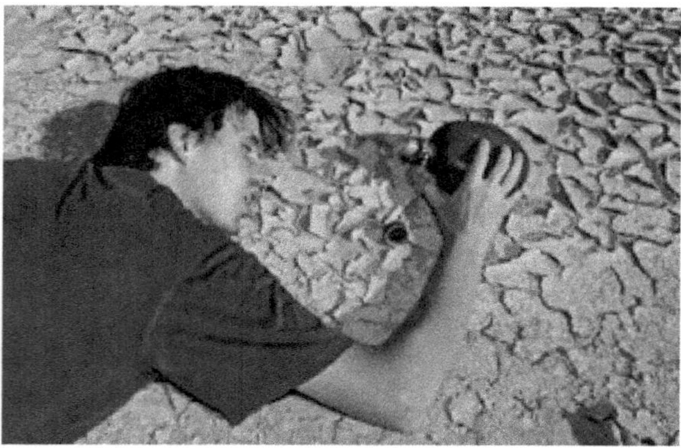

If you possess limited amount of water, then you must avoid eating. If the temperature is above than 38-degree C then you must drink at least one liter water after every 60 minutes. And if the temperature is below than 38-degree C then try to drink at least half liter water after every sixty seconds.

Skill #14-Bearing the Tropical Weather

General concept is that surviving in the Tropical region is extremely difficult as it mainly consists of dense rain forests, which in fact is not true. Surviving in tropical area is not as difficult as you will have variety of options to fulfill your basic necessities for food, shelter and safety.

If we talk about the weather conditions of the tropical region then yes they are really tough, because the weather in this area is totally unpredictable. The temperatures are quite high during the day plus the excessive humidity makes it extremely difficult to breathe in this region. If you are residing in the areas located at the height of around 15000 meters then you must brace yourself for the chilling cold at night time.

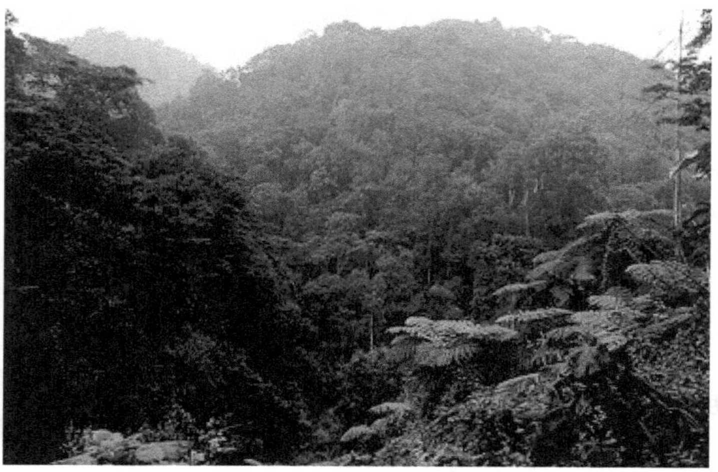

https://www.arborday.org/programs/rainforest/report/2011/images/rain-forest-lg.jpg

During the rains, the temperature will go down and the environment will become pleasant but after the rain stops, the temperature will again rise to the unbearable height. The rainfall is quite heavy and can cause hurricanes so in order avoid any damage from the storm, you must make a careful selection of your shelter.

Skill #15-Fighting the Cold

If you got stuck in the cold mountainous area then the first thing you must do is to gain as much knowledge about your surroundings and weather conditions of that area as possible. One of the biggest issues of the cold areas is the wind-chill that will bump into your body whenever you move around. Another big issue is to find a suitable warm shelter and food items in the cold areas.

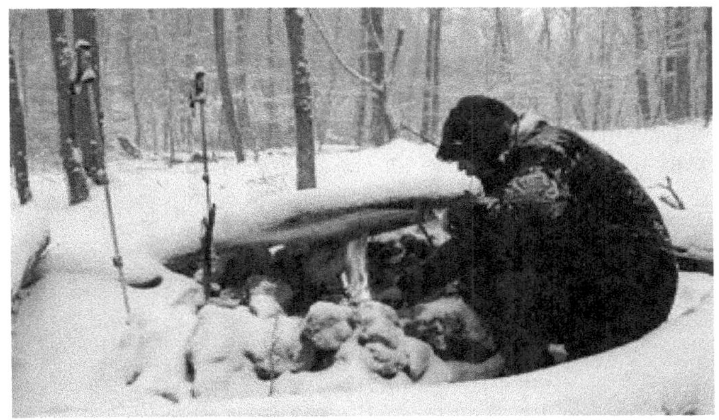

http://www.thebugoutbagguide.com/wp-content/uploads/2014/02/Cold-Weather-Survival2.jpg

You must have sufficient warm clothes so keep you hot. And mind it that you must always wear clean clothes during the chilling cold otherwise your clothes will not be able to protect you. You must also possess a strong will-power in order to fight with the severities of the cold areas otherwise you won't be able to survive.

Skill #16-Keeping Yourself Alive in the Sea

While in the sea, you can face various life-threatening situations such as excessive heat or excessive cold. In such conditions, you must keep your mind present and make careful use of the resources that are available to you at the time. If due to any reason you have fallen into the open sea then you must know the strategies to swim in the most comfortable way possible.

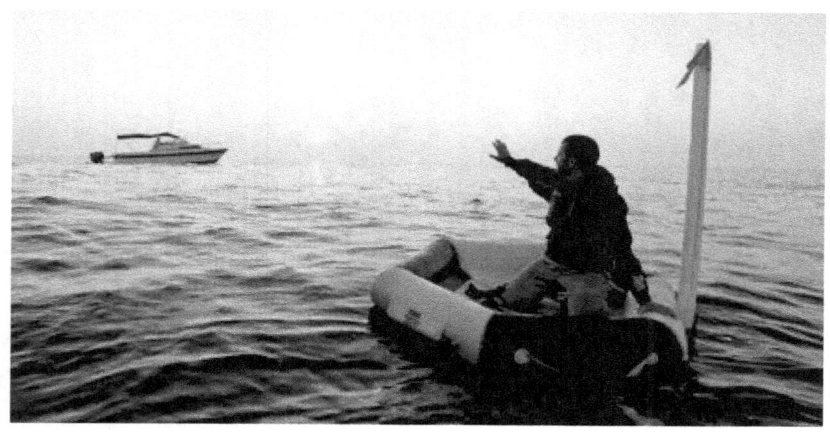

http://patriotrising.com/wp-content/uploads/2014/07/survive-sea.jpg

Skill #17-Surviving the Water Crossings

While dwelling in the wilderness, you might have to cross a river or a lake someday. So in order to cross it safely, you must have a complete knowledge of the precautionary measures that you must follow while crossing it. Before entering the water, you must first remove your clothes so the weight of the water won't affect your movements. You must secure your survival kit on your shoulders and hold a long stick to find your way safely into the water. Your stick must be strong and around 2.5 meters long so it can go far-deep under the water.

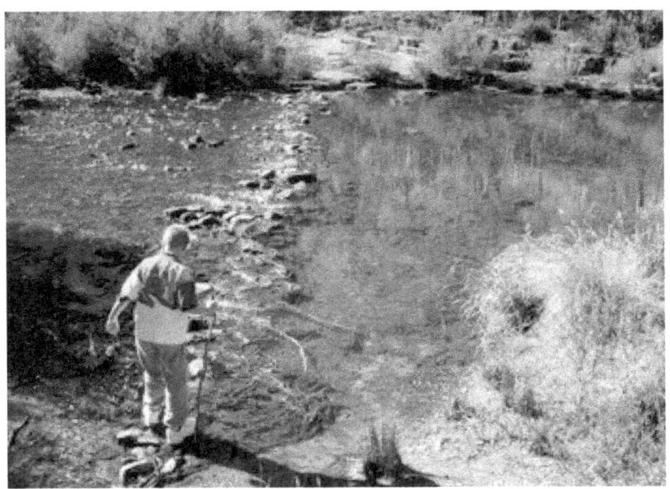

http://www.gmilburn.ca/wp-content/uploads/2010/11/river-crossing.jpg

Skill #18- Finding Your Way in the Wilderness

While staying in the wilderness, you might have to walk far-away from your shelter in order to find food and water. You can also get lost in such a situation. So you must know the strategies to find your way back to your shelter. You can determine the directions with the help of the sun.

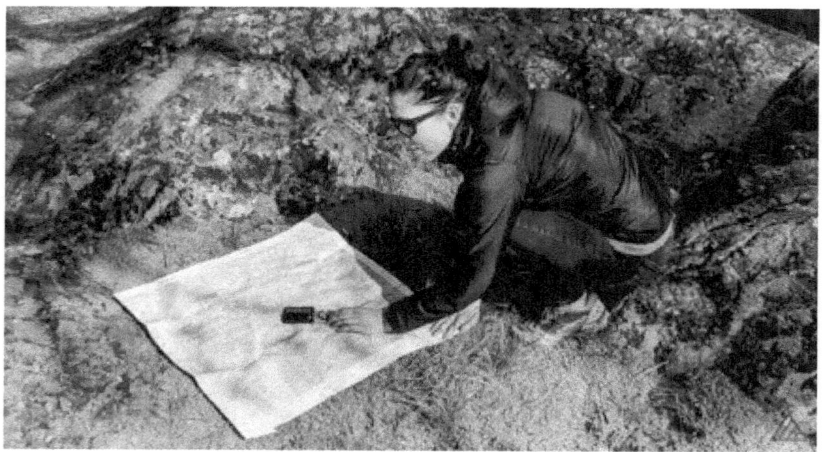

https://www.mbguiding.ca/wp-content/uploads/2016/03/wilderness-navigation-map-compass-demo-1200x675.jpg

Usually sun sets in the west but rises in the east. But in fact these directions are not too accurate as sun slightly changes its rising and setting destinations according to the seasons and movements of the earth.

You can also use the moon and the stars method to find the directions.

Skill #19-Crying for help

Getting rescued from the wilderness is the only hope that a person can have. But what are methods through which we can cry for help? You can create some physical signals lying around such as pieces of your clothing, or a watch.

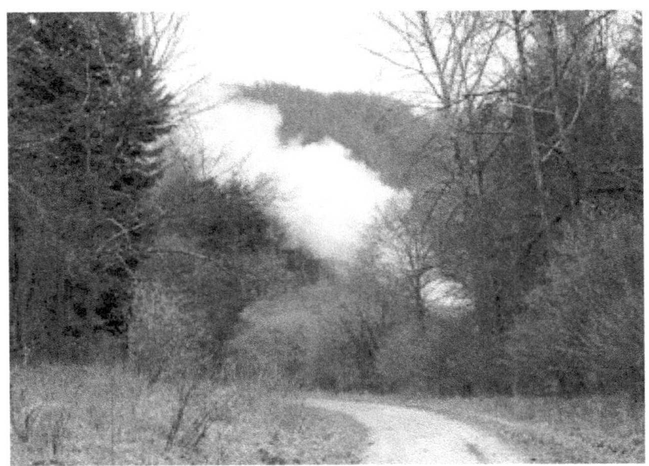

You can also light huge fire in order to signal for help through the smoke or you can also burn a tree.

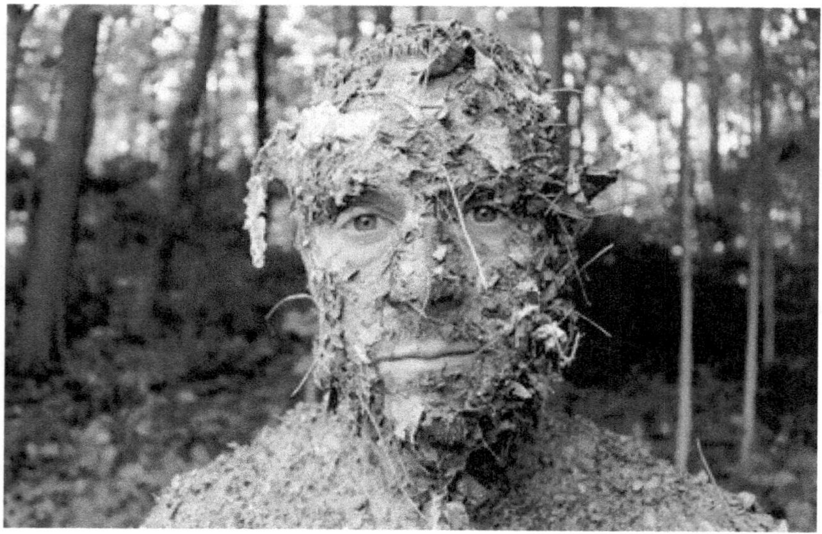

http://tipsforsurvivalists.com/wp-content/uploads/2014/07/creek-stewart-face.jpg

You have created a shelter, you managed to find food and water, you also signaled for help, now the last thing is to keep yourself safe and alive till the help arrives for you. The only way to stay alive is to camouflage yourself, your equipment and your shelter. You can pick items out of your surroundings to blend in with your environment.

Conclusion

You might never know when you suddenly fall into a situation where you have to fight for survival in the wilderness. This book is a must-read for every person whether he/she likes to go on adventurous trips or not. Surviving in the wilderness is not a piece of cake as you have to face many hardships. After reading this book you will definitely be able to handle any such situation if and when it arises.

During your reading journey of this book, you have learnt how to find and create a safe shelter, how to find food items, how to distinguish between poisonous food items and safe food items, how to find the drinking water, how to create weapons from your surroundings and how to keep yourself alive. After reading all these chapters, you must have gained sufficient knowledge for the tactics to survive while residing in the wilderness.

Special thanks to you for downloading this informative book as this book contains information on one of the most important topics of life. Apart from learning the 20 helpful skills mentioned in this book, you must keep your will-power extremely strong. Because if a person possesses strong will-power then he can easily fight with the biggest hurdles of this world but if the will-power is not strong then he can't keep himself alive even if the circumstances are not so hard. Apart from keeping strong will-power, a person must keep his mind present and not panic when a sudden calamity befalls him.

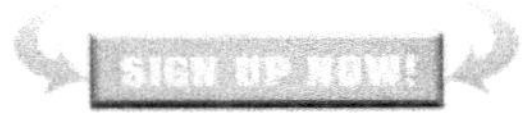

OR Go to this URL

http://zbit.ly/1WBb1Ek